POEMS
to
Encourage
and
INSPIRE

JANICE E. MANNEX

Ordering Information:

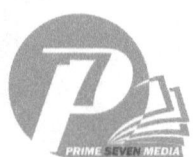

Prime Seven Media
518 Landmann St.
Tomah City, WI 54660

Printed in the United States of America

Common English Bible

New International Version UK

TABLE OF CONTENTS

VOLUME 1

Acknowledgements

I would like to acknowledge and thank all those who have encouraged me to publish the poetry God inspires me to write.

I especially wish to acknowledge my sister Irene Hopkins who gifted me the lovely photo "Mount Taranaki" to use on the front cover.

To *www.Biblegateway.com* for having a website that made adding the scripture verses I wanted so easy.

What God has done in my life.

God first looked after me when I was born to loving parents on 9th January 1954.

He ensured even though mum and dad had clashing blood types I only got mild after effects mentioned below. (Many babies were severely disabled or died before birth with the RH negative factor in those days.)

2 ½ years later He gave mum the strength to carry on and do a good job raising my sister and me when dad died 8 months after contracting Polio

He helped me through school especially the early years when I was teased both for a speech impediment and co-ordination problems

He ensured I got speech help at primary school. I hated this as a 7 to 9 year old! As I often would miss out on class swimming time because of speech. Speech consisted of learning many poems and rhyming jingles. As always God knew what He was doing ; 50 years in the future He'd use this for His work!

Mum ensured we attended Sunday School and when I was about 13 at a Presbyterian Easter Camp in Eltham, Taranaki I gave my life to Him.

He ensured I was accepted and passed my Community Nursing course and gave me a passion for the elderly and significantly disabled.

In 1985 I fell in love and got married

God upheld, loved and often carried me through the next 17 years.

In early 1986 I became pregnant with our first son and we were really excited.

Late October the specialist told me (when I was alone) at an antenatal appointment that there was a problem with my babies brain. I would probably have to have a Cesaerian Section and baby would be 6 weeks premature and may be severely disabled and not live!

The paediatricians had other ideas and my precious son was carried to 38 weeks and while John has some significant disabilities God ensured I did not have a dead baby but a precious loving son.

Praise God for giving the plumber whose own baby had hydrocephalus the skills to design the first shunt to bypass the blockage. Without this dad thousands of babies world- wide would not have lived over the previous 20 years including John!

God carried me supporting me with Christian Music and Poetry while John went through 17 lots of brain surgery in his first 7 years of life Including when John was about 18 months my marriage broke up due to my husband but not admitting he wasn't coping with the continued stress of John's medical problems.

When John was about 15 he caught a very bad virus and lost heaps of weight, no doctor thought to check his blood medication levels and one level got far too high this caused him to become extremely violent without warning. God carried me giving me the wisdom to do a very difficult thing for any mother; to place John in care for my own and his 13 yrs old brothers safety.

In November 2006 I was listening to Life FM in the car one morning before going in to teacher aide the very high needs student I was working with, when I heard the quote *"If God takes you to it He will get you through it"* and thought to myself gee that will be really useful to share one day.

Under 36 hours later I was the one needing that quote to help me through God's timing always perfect!

Contact had always been maintained with John and 2 years later God kept his brother and me safe when John came home for a two hour visit and due to things earlier in the day John lost it putting James and my lives in danger for a short period.

During this period God prompted me to follow John's brother and change churches to attend City West Church where I could worship without well-meaning people asking how John was. Amazing the difference this made and I found a much greater depth to my relationship with my Lord.

God gave me the wisdom to see through my feelings and make the decision that John could never visit again unless accompanied by staff.

That night I cried out to My Lord what am I to do now ?

Next morning, I awoke still feeling shattered WHEN... the room suddenly became full of God's peace.

I thought I was ready for what He was going to tell me to do,

BUT I CERTAINLY WAS NOT EXPECTING WHAT HE SAID TO ME!!

As soon as I was soaking up His peace God said to me

"You are to sell this place and move out to live with and care for your mother, for me" I replied asking him "what was that last part, Lord?" He replied "you heard me, you can do it, act quickly. You are to move by the start of the school year" Several friends and extended family told me: "it won't work," "she'll break you" "you can't do it" **BUT** For the first time in my life I knew emphatically the devil was trying to derail my life and God's plan.

Ignoring all the comments I obeyed God. The house sold quickly before being put on the market ; for the required amount God's confirmation to me. To say the next few months were trying is a major understatement. But with God's helping hand, we made it through.

Women's conference 08: God gave me 3 messages. Go through the waters of baptism, tell your story, I am all and more than you need My water baptism in July 08 Again the devil tried to derail this. I woke with an asthma attack that day which should have seen me in A & E not at church. No way was I missing my baptism, using heaps of ventolin to get there. God's awesome response HE removed troublesome asthma from my life that night.

Only a few months later I was baptised in the Holy Spirit and God turned up massively the speed on the escalator of growth in my Christian faith. Within weeks a Christian friend who didn't know about it asked me what had changed. She said."You have so much confidence, you are sharing openly what has changed ?"

God really ignited a passion to get Christian Poetry recorded and out there on CD at this stage and a few weeks later a friend challenged me to write some of my own. The very next day God gave me the words to my first poem. In the last two years God has:

- Healed 25yr old injuries to my neck and shoulder ligaments.
- Prompted me to get over my technophobia and start using technology to share the poetry he inspires me to write. *www.life-poetry-to-encourage.com* is a direct result of obedience to this instruction.
- He continues to challenge, stretch and look after me. Enabling me to bless others by sharing His unconditional love for everyone through my poetry

God is waiting and wanting to look after you, He has always loved you ; in turn using you to spread His good word.
God Bless Janice Mannex

Fear Not

Satan's fear has no power when
We travel through life with Jesus at our side

So boldly step out and fear not,
When tough, life has got
God has given us such a lot.

Be aware but don't despair
Satan's always very near
Ready to instil into you…A spirit of fear

There's just no room
For Satan's fear
To give you a wild ride
When daily we have Jesus alongside.

This master of trickery and disguise
Cannot succeed when we keep
Jesus close by our side.

Jesus, is our guide
The letters of that word fear
Stand for what we have to lean on
With Jesus at our side.

F is for	Faithful friend
E is for	Everlasting encourager
A is for	Awesome anchor
R is for	Rescuing redeemer.

Reach out and grasp Jesus's hand
He will bury Satan's fear deep down in the very hot sand
Restoring your confidence so, you again will feel grand.

Remember
Jesus is always our
Faithful friend
Everlasting encourager
Awesome anchor
Rescuing redeemer

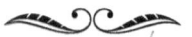

Genesis 15 :1 The Message
"After all these things this word of God came unto Abram in a vision:
"Don't be afraid Abram: I 'm your shield, Your reward will be grand.""

This poem was written one week following an awful situation I went through on the preceding Tuesday. In the wee small hours of the morning God gave me these words and through these words both reassured me and reminded me that He had a purpose for it; and would be using the strength and insight I gained from clinging onto Him in it for His work in the future. May it be a blessing to all those who read it.

When Upon Life's Journey

When upon Life's journey, You do find
You are in places not very kind
Remember as far fetched as it may seem
Right here and now
God planned your life's journey
He had this in His mind

To equip you to be His vessel
Pouring out His love, His peace, His kindness,
No matter what situation you find
For evermore.

With His love and His grace
He will ensure you safely complete life's race
Arriving at Heaven's door with many more
That know & love Him because you were His vessel
Pouring out His love, His peace, His kindness
Whenever, wherever you came across
Those in situations… that were not very kind.

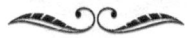

Jeremiah 29:11 (CEB)
*   **11** I know the plans I have in mind for you, declares the Lord; they are plans for peace, not disaster, to give you a future filled with hope.*

Inspired by our Lord through a message on how not all God's promises are that everything will be good and easy; but that He will bring us through safely and Never Ever leave us alone.

His Promises

Many promises God gave us, are to help us, through life.
Including times, of, real strife.
He didn't promise a fairy tale ride
Instead… He'd, be there for us when, life's a wild ride!

When, through dark pathways our life is creeping,
Satan sometimes, tricks us into thinking;
Our Saviour… is not His own promises keeping!

Never ever, is that true.
God knows each one of us through and through.

Press into Jesus at those times He'll encourage and guide you,
Helping you, to make it through.

Fall not, into Satan's sneaky traps,
Pressing the buttons pause, delete or rewind
The fast forward button is what Our Lord had in mind.
Leading, each one of us along our special pathway
Till on reaching our heavenly home those pearly gates we enter

Deuteronomy 31:8 KJV
*"And the Lord, He it is that doth go before Thee. He will be with Thee.
He will not fail Thee, neither forsake Thee: Fear not neither be dismayed"*

This poem was inspired by a rainbow that appeared in the very threatening looking sky while doing a fundraising BBQ for a local Christian radio station. It started a conversation on what rainbows meant to us personally between myself and the other helper at the time.

His Rainbows

The beauty of… Our Heavenly Father's creation,
The reminder of… His promises are easy for us to see.
Whenever skies are stormy,
He places beautiful rainbows in the sky.

When times in life are stormy
I need only to remember Him
Picturing His beautiful rainbows.
Asking Him to provide me
The help, reassurance & confidence.

Lots of people seek mystical pots of gold
Said to be found at the rainbows end
Instead… of turning…
To the one and only… true pot of gold
God's love, which never ever comes to an end.

His glorious rainbows reminding me,
He is the great creator,
His promises are everlasting,
And are always readily available to me.

So,
when you wish, . . . you were lucky,
Already holding, that mystical pot of gold, in your hands
Call out to Our Heavenly Father
He always hears, everyone
And He never turns anyone down!

FOR He's ready to help you
HE knows and understands
Just what you need... right at that moment.
His patience, waiting for your call lasts indefinitely.
His love for you is above and beyond all
IT WILL NEVER EVER COME TO AN END!!

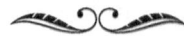

Genesis 9 :12-15 (Common English Bible)
*   **12** God said, "This is the symbol of the covenant that I am drawing up between me and you and every living thing with you, on behalf of every future generation. **13** I have placed my bow in the clouds; it will be the symbol of the covenant between me and the earth. **14** When I bring clouds over the earth and the bow appears in the clouds, **15** I will remember the covenant between me and you and every living being among all the creatures.*

The following poem inspired by reassurances from God after a very trying, day long situation caring for someone.

Part of His Plan

Sometimes life just don't seem fair
Full of hurts worries and cares
But don't despair there is a reason
Tis only one of Gods seasons.

Seasons placed strategically
Growing us until
We tell others enthusiastically
How He never ever fails to care
When we call out to Him in prayer.

His timing, His ways, we don't understand
Yet certain we can be… He's in control
And… It is all part of His special master plan.

It's many years late
We recognise the part it had to play
Enabling us, to be able to do His work today.

"God's name is a place of protection—good people can run there and be safe"

Proverbs 18.10 (The Message)

This poem my Lord gave me the words to as I drove to my friends place for a day away from a stressful situation at the time. It is the first poem He ever enabled me to write and was the day after my friend had challenged me to write some of my own.

Life's Hurdles

Since time begun,
And we were young.
Life's hurdles, a many have come.

Without warning they come,
But do not fret, to our aid when young,
Mum or dad come.

As older we get,
Harder hurdles God sets,

But do not forget!
Jesus, Our Lord,
To our aid always comes,
If only,
we'll ask Him to help us overcome.

Luke1:37(NIV UK)
    "For nothing is impossible with God"

This poem is a reflection of how God looked after me during the very tough years after my disabled sons birth.

Troubles

When life's troubles are too massive a task,
He'll catch you!
Along the troubled pathway,
He'll carry you !
When it seems too hard to keep going,
He'll cradle you!
When He calls loved ones home,
He'll comfort you!

Jesus cares, He's always here
Catching, carrying, Cradling, and comforting
All those who ask Him.

Looking back, glimpses He's given me of;
Where He's caught me, When He's carried me,
Where He's cradled me, When He's comforted me.

Where He's caught you, When He's carried you,
Where He's cradled you, When He's comforted you.
Will be plain to see, When at last life's work is done
And
He's called you home to sit on His knee.

Onward I go, though trouble and woe
May visit me.
I know, He's always there,
And one day, I'll sit on His knee
My Jesus and me!

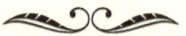

Hebrews 13:5(The Message)

*Don't be obsessed with getting more material things. Be relaxed with what **you** have. Since God assured us, "**I'll never** let **you** down, **never** walk off and **leave you**," we can boldly quote, God is there, ready to help; **I'm** fearless no matter what. Who **or** what can get to me?*

*Inspired by the different pathways and degrees of steepness &
speed of them God takes each of us on to continue His good work
right on time.*

The Staircase

Lord Jesus
A staircase you've set for us to climb
No other is the same as mine
Each staircase You designed especially
To enable us to climb it successfully.
Each step requires the best from us
Daily asking for Your help a must!
Landings a plenty, You put in place
So we can rest then, renew the pace

When at last we reach the top
Heaven's doors will open pop.

And You will say home
You're here to stay.

Psalm23 :1-3 (The Message)
God, my shepherd! I don't need a thing.
You have bedded me down in lush meadows,
You find me quiet pools to drink from.
True to your word,

You let me catch my breath
and send me in the right direction.

Written after My Lord had kept me securely walking with Him and caring for mum. Satan had tried to derail this through a support service review. Prayer support kept me calm and thinking logically and praising Our Lord and with Him Satan has been defeated!! Thank You Lord!

Jesus Our Rock

Jesus is our rock,
When in Him we stand
He will gently guide us, along the road He's planned

For He has promised
Always to hold our hand
Even when… we don't understand!
How life right now… can be part of His plan!

You can always be very sure
He will never let go of your precious hand

So securely anchor your feet, onto Jesus your rock
His hand into yours firmly lock

Satan then trying as hard as he can
Will not… successfully your walk, with your Lord unlock.
Never ever, will Satan, be able to drag you
Down, to his very hot sandy land.

Isaiah 28 v 16 NIV
   "so this is what the Sovereign Lord says" See, I lay a stone in Zion, a tested stone. A precious cornerstone for a sure foundation. The one who relies on it will never be stricken with panic"

I was inspired to write this poem while reflecting on how He has enabled me to carry on giving out day after day for over two months now while in several situations My Lord needed me to show His Love and care to close friends and extended family.

My Lord

God is my Heavenly Father!
Jesus Christ is my Lord!
In wonder I will praise Him!
In thanks I'll always honour Him!
Forever I will serve Him!

For He guides me
Each and every step of the way
He helps me not to stray
He gives me strength to do His work;
Each and every day

He provides grace for the work
He has for me each day
He provides peace to settle,
Human emotions within
So through me; He can shine
Such amazing, unending love
That can only come from Him

When I grow weary in a trial
Wondering how much more
I can give Him my best

He encourages me
through that trial
He finds a way to give me a rest
Lord, others different skills you've given
Enabling still others to impart
the love and care You send from Heaven
on Your behalf.
Jesus Christ My Lord and Saviour
YOU ARE THE VERY BEST!!!!!!

Psalm 23:3 (GNT)
    "He gives me new strength;He guides me in the right paths as He has promised."

This is very much what Our Lord means to me; and reflects things He has done for me in my life. Written after my special lad asked me to write a poem to help him through "some humps I have to get over here." verses 4 &5 have wording special to John in them.

Lord You Are

Lord, You are my light,
Shining down on me.
Helping me, to do things right,
By showing me the way.
Turning hard times, into nice days.

Lord, You are my guide,
Guiding me from above,
Whispering instructions, quietly with love.

Lord, You are my strength,
Telling me to step out,
Without any doubt.
Not to fear, as You are always there.

Lord, You are my comforter,
When I need it most,
Your loving arms are there for me.
Giving me a cuddle,
So I'm no longer in a stressed muddle
Lord, . . . You are my helper
When times are tough
You... Help me to keep my cool

Lord, You are my teacher
With you as teacher, I can achieve
Far beyond my wildest dreams.

Lord, You are my carer
Your care for me. Is more than I need
SO
I can care for others increasingly more
Like You care for me.

Lord Jesus, You are everything to me!
Thank you for being who you are!!

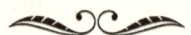

Psalm 62:2
    He alone is my rock and my salvation; He is my fortress, I will never be shaken."

A reflection on a coach that never gives up Our Lord Jesus Christ

Supercoach

Life is a steeplechase,
Many hurdles we'll face.
Live it, Like it's
An important race.

These hurdles we face
Are put in place
To continue to grow us
Using His wonderful grace

Another stage of lifes' steeplechase is done
When through His help that hurdle is overcome

No matter how much, how often we muck up
Jesus is ready to pick us up
Whenever, we ask Him for a hand up.

Picked up and restored
He sets us back at the right place
On life's steeplechase track.

Jesus, our coach will never quit,
Not even, when the finish line we hit.
Welcoming us to our Heavenly home
Life's steeplechase here on Earth, Successfully won.

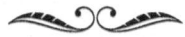

Mathew 28.20 (The Message)
"I will be with you as you do this day after day, right up to the end of the age."

Inspiration for this poem came from a speaker who shared her testimony at a conference

He's Our Recycler

Lord,
You rescue us from strife
You encourage others through struggles in life

You comfort us when times are tough
Bearing our yoke when… it is too much

You confirm, Your love whenever we falter
You lead us through trials
Enabling us to lead others to You

You are the Everlasting Supporter,
You are the Ultimate Redeemer
You are the Greatest Recycler

Our
Rescuing,
Encouraging
Comforting
Yoke bearing
Confirming
Leading
Everlasting
Redeeming Saviour and Friend.

Psalms 103:12 (The Message)
   "As far as sunrise is from sunset He has separated us from our sins."

This poem was written after a guest speaker at a women's conference urged us to be alert for ways we can show God's and love and care everywhere, every day of the week

Opportunities

Lord, opportunities you give us
Everyday… Anywhere
To show the world
How to care and how to love Your way.

The opportunities that you give us Lord
To show your care, to show your love
May only take us a second to give
That much needed wave or smile
Or may take us quite a while.

The opportunities that you give Lord
Maybe obvious for all to see
OR Maybe only to be seen by me.
Lord
Help us all to do your work everywhere we go
Not to be blind to any opportunity
To show Your care, to show Your love to all folks everywhere.

Mathew25:40(NIV UK)
"The king will reply. "I tell you the truth, whatever you did for one of the least of these brothers of mine, you did for me."

I was working on editing my Christian Poetry website one morning and was having some technical problems. I went to set up a page to test if something was corrected and had to name the page "Trials" was instantly there. Over the next hour as I worked on the site I repeatedly got prompted to pen a poem on the subject; below is the poem.

Trials

Trials come and trials go,
Why we may not ever know
At times we want to turn away
Maybe to come back another day
Or, go completely the other way.
Technology and me often disagree

Then Satan rubs His hands in glee
Hoping, I'll now go his way!
Never will I turn that way
Jesus is the way for me!

Trials are sent from God above
One at a time, so we can cope
Bringing us closer to Him and His perfect love

Jesus first through them had to go
So He could show us the way through
With Jesus, our guide we will survive
Finding, our way each and every day
Heavenly Father, thank You.

Psalm 18:28-30 (NIV)

You, Lord, keep my lamp burning; my God turns my darkness into light. With Your help I can advance against a troop; with my God I can scale a wall. As for God, his way is perfect: The Lord's word is flawless; He shields all who take refuge in Him."

Inspired, by messages at church the two last Sunday nights, reminding us God needs us to do all the things he asks of us. God will never ask us to do anything that with His help we cannot complete.

Don't Sit On The Bench

Who, me coach? I am not good enough to play
You sure don't want me on the field today
I'll just sit on the bench and watch this game
Cheering, my teammates onto fame.

Half time came and went,
Right down to the wire that game went
When the full time arrived… every ounce
of energy had been spent
By those, who obeyed the coach that day.

Extra time needed to be played
Who would win the game that day?
Your team so tired… they did not find,
the energy needed for extra time
Your team that day found no fame.,
They did not win that game
Was it because you chose not to play?

Jesus our coach… asks us to step up to the plate
To do the special things… He's there in wait
So don't sit on the bench. Don't be slow to step up
Our Heavenly Fathers work still needs to be done,
There are many more lives for Him to be won.

Ephesians 2:10

Instead, we are God's accomplishment, created in Christ Jesus to do **good** *things. God planned for these* **good** *things to be the way that we live our lives.*

This poem was written after a friend recalled to me how in several periods of despair when she called out help to our Lord suddenly she was aware of encouraging people surrounding her.

Just call on our Lord

No matter, what the circumstance
No matter, what the fear
No matter, if it's big or small

Our Lord will help us overcome them all
Whenever, we remember to give Him a call.

So, boldly step forward
Without any worries, without any doubt

Lord, when our pleas on Your ears do fall,
You've already got our help in place
Just waiting for us on You to call.

Then, from deep despair
We suddenly find encouraging people everywhere
Visiting us or… Upholding us through prayer.

Earlier, of their presence we were totally unaware.
So always give Our Lord a shout
He will always help you out!
Lord
So awesome, is Your wonderful grace,
No matter what circumstance we face.!!

Psalm56 :3
   "when ever I am afraid I will put my trust in you"

This poem was written after I was realized God's purpose for situations that I certainly could not see at the time could possibly be His doing.

God Never Disappears

God never disappears.
Although at times It seems
He's not there!

He's always waiting,
Ready, with His wonderful care.
For us, to tell Him
Life's getting hard to bear.

When,
We send Him a help please prayer.
You can be sure He will hear
AND
He will on you,
Pour out His Loving care!

Joshua 1:5 (The Message)
"In the same way I was with Moses, I'll be with you. I won't give up on you; I won't leave you."

This poem was written after hearing a message at a conference on keeping His fire alive and ready in our hearts and also reflecting on two Sunday school favourite hymns ; Jesus Bids Us Shine and Hide It Under A Bushel, NO!

Beacons in the Night

We are called to be a beacon
Showing others the way
So that, they in turn… can find their way,
When skies above their path
Are dark, and stormy grey.

With His fire in our hearts
We are a beacon in the dark.
Feed this fire day and night
Keep that beacon, shining bright.

To be His beacons in the night
We must… be sure…
His Fire… in us, Is burning bright.

We must carry God's fire on each hill we climb
As on, the next hilltop we may find
His fire refuelled and ready Is needed to ensure,
Everybody there remains just fine.

When life's journey, for us is not easy
And the flames within grow dim
Strengthen the fire by asking Him
Lord,
Please re-ignite Your Holy Fire within.

Then the fire in us, again will be,
The bright guiding light, Jesus intended it to be.
Strong and beautiful Like He.

Matthew 5: 15
"If I make you light bearers, you don't think I'm going to hide you under a bucket, do you? I'm putting you on a light stand- Shine! The Message

This poem was written to show and encourage others to look back and see how The Lord supports us through situations by using people, events etc we certainly wouldn't have expected to be part of the solution.

His Unexpected Way

In need of a rest, I asked our Lord,
Where O where, would I somehow find
Mother friendly, relief care?

Jesus sent my son, unemployed temporarily
Home to live with mother and me.

Only Jesus could see
How a rest that could be.
But a refreshing rest it just happened to be

My son's new job starting precisely when
my sister was again able to assist me.

So be prepared with eyes open to see
The unexpected ways He answers your pleas
His timing perfect will be
His care always there.

Jesus knows, He has already planned
What assistance we'll receive
When we request Him to assist
He's so pleased.

Thank you Lord,
You answered my heartfelt plea.
Thank you for the unexpected way.
You refreshed me.

Luke 11: 9 &10 (The Message)
"Here's what I am saying: Ask and you'll get;Seek and you'll find;
Knock and the door will open."

Written leading up to Easter. I was reflecting on Our Heavenly Fathers awesome creation : BUT how much more awesome the gift of His Son going to Calvary and setting us free was.

Reflection of Calvary

My mind is set on Calvary
Of the magnificent gift, that there took place
My eyes, are locked on the face
Of Jesus… my rock.

On that lovely autumn morning
As up our track, I walked
I was totally in awe… of God's magnificent creation.

My gaze was locked
Onto Taranaki's big rock
Mount Egmont,
As I know it from way back

Supremely beautiful
majestic and clear
Its rocky slopes almost bare
In… our crisp autumn air.
Sprinkled… down from its' crown
Were… remnants of the regions' first snow.

Suddenly... It dawned on me
The picture... that snow was making
Was... Of His blood
Trickling down His face
From... that thorny crown... Christ wore for us
At Calvary.

Only... it was white
Signifying... the new pure life
For which... He so freely gave
His life.

Releasing you and me
From sin
Forever... To be free.

Now... forever
Mt Egmont will be
A daily reminder to me
Of the cost... at the Cross of Calvary
And what it means to me.

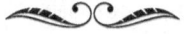

Mark 16:16 (NIV)

Don't be alarmed" he said "You are looking for Jesus the Nazarene who was crucified, He has risen! He is not here. See the place they laid Him."

The inspiration for this poem came as I saw the perfection in the coat of snow on Mt Taranaki last winter BUT God prompted me it was not complete until this morning when I woke up and He had me add one line to it and change one other word

Clean As Snow

At crack of dawn, One winters morn
My eyes were drawn
To a heavily and snow clad mountain.

Proudly displaying
A coat of fresh new snow
so perfectly complete.

All, not quite right was hidden from sight
as if it never existed before.

When to Jesus on our knees we humbly go
He will completely wash us,
So we become pure and complete
just like that coat of snow.

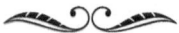

Psalm 51:7 (GNT)
   "Remove my sin, and I will be clean; Wash me, and I will be whiter than snow."

The following poem was inspired by God using advanced medical technology to restore health to two very precious children close to our family against all odds! Praise Him! Showing me also how much general and prayer support from across the world was made possible through the Internet and social media sites. That He wanted me to embrace modern technology more making the poetry He enables me to write available to so many more people.

Technology It is Part of His Plan!!!

Technology is advancing at such a pace
To everyday people it seems
just like Inventors are in a pointless mad race.
Everyday people unsure Lord
If it's something they want to embrace.

The pace of this race exists to allow
You, Lord to show
Your Love, Your Care and Your Grace
When circumstances in Your perfect plan
Would otherwise be too hard
For Your people to face.

Lord, You gave everyday people
Skills… needed to invent and design.
The technology You had in mind,
That needed to completed
by everyday man… exactly on time.

So, each vital step in Your plan was already in place
Allowing You Lord to once again show us, just everyday people
Your Love Your care and Your Grace

Technology that unites friends, families and workmates
From all over the Earth enabling them to support
Everyday people, going through strife.

Gone are the days of painful hospital corridor queues
Everyday people waiting to use the one and only payphone
To contact those that, anxiously wait at home
For someone to call with the daily news.

The Internet, is just part of that race
Instantly enabling Christians to unite
Supporting each other with messages of Your Love
To those whose needs it fits like a glove.

Medical technology, another area Lord,
advancing at race like pace.
Enabling Doctors and Surgeons to show
Your Love, Your Care and Your Grace
Saving and improving more lives every day of every year.

Social Media and other technology
mistakes are all we seem to hear
Everyday people, then slow to embrace
technology that enables them to share
Your Love, Your Care and Your Grace everywhere.

Help us Lord, to not hinder Your plan
By getting entrapped and holding back
From embracing at pace technology that enables us to share
Your Grace, Your Love and Your Care.

Jeremiah 29:11
For I know the plans I have for you," declares the LORD, "plans to prosper you and not to harm you, plans to give you hope and a future." NIV

This poem was written to encourage a new Christian friend who was going through a tough time.

Don't Give Up

Don't give up… cheer up
Keep plodding on
Day after day for Jesus
You can be sure that
Jesus will always help you to keep plodding on.

Never a prayer He forgets
But He waits.
Answering them in His perfect time
So His plan for us He can complete
With His ultimate loving care.

In His time… your cup will overflow
That is when Our Lord answers
All the prayers from long ago
You sent Him, every single one!

Inspired to write this while my church pastors were spending a few services with messages based on points raised in the book "The15 challenge

Just Do It

Jesus asks us… to take time out
To help someone else
Along their way each day.

Busy lives are filled with this and that
Are you thinking
Wherever, whenever & however
Will I fit in that.?
Jesus provides the opening
When we are ready to give out
His love entering our hearts
Like a jet engines blast.

The thrust, created just enough
So we give out just what is needed
When and where the need is.

Someone there, you can be sure
Will, later on, seek His love and grace
Totally unknown to them,
it was before, You stepped out in faith… And went to their door.

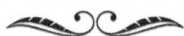

Luke 10 36-37 (The Message)
"what do you think? Which of the three became a neighbour to the man attacked by robbers?" "The one who treated him kindly", the religion scholar responded. Jesus said, "Go and do the same."

This poem is the end result of a sermon one Sunday night, on missions not only being overseas. It really spoke to me and before I could go to sleep that night; I had to write down the message God had given me through it.

Mission Fields

Spread my good news,
By thought word and deed
Our Saviour said.
So all peoples can be led,
and the beggars can be fed.

Mission work for me, Oh No!,
Overseas travel was all I could see
And it certainly was not for me!!

When I opened my eyes to see what He sees
Mission fields nearby never seen before
Were very clear to see.

Schools, friends, workmates and others we meet
What about the people in the house across the street?

My own community, and places I go
The mission fields shown to me.
So open your eyes to see as He sees
Then your mission fields
Clear to you will be.

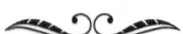

Mark 16:15 (The Message)
   "Go into the world, go everywhere and announce the Message of God's good news to one and all."

Poem inspired by a visiting preachers message on being sure we do not take off God's armour even when we are asleep.

Our Lord Is Able

Our Lord is able to do anything
Fill, any canyon, mend, any hurt.

Victorious over troubles is He
When openly, His assistance seek we.
He will, for you, win the victory.

Put on God's armour, wear it day and night.
Train yourself ready for the spiritual fight
Then, You, will win that fight.

Satan is trouble with a capital T
Very sneaky and convincing is he.

So fill up your spiritual fuel tank,
Retrain yourself continually.

And you will, with Our Lord
Have the victory.

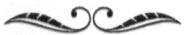

Mark 10:27 NIV©2011
'Jesus looked at them and said "with man this is impossible, but not with God; all things are possible with God"'

The inspiration for this short poem was a bible verse used at a pre service prayer meeting.

Jesus Our Restorer

Jesus restores us
When our trust we put in Him
Even, when that trust is weak and mighty thin.

He restores everything be it big or small
Hurts, grief and relationships,
To name just a few. He restores them all
So don't make a big fuss
Just get on that prayer bus
And tell them all to Him.

2 Corinthians 5:18
*All of these **new things** are from God, who reconciled us to himself through Christ and who gave us the ministry of reconciliation.*

Our Lord inspired this poem after the first earthquake. I was praising Him at the time for no fatalities and praying for all the families in Christchurch

The Quakes

Early in the morning,
Most people sound asleep.

When, all of a sudden
The land started to shake.
What a mess, it was going to make!

Aftershocks by the hundreds,
Rubble piles by the score.
When O when
Are they going to stop shaking the door?

Severity and damage so grand,
Putting fear and trauma,
Into lives, across our land.

God's reasons for this shaky season,
We don't understand.
Was it… To shake us awake,
A better nation,
Of us, to make?

No loss of life, few badly hurt.
A clear sign
God is still at work.
Defending, the people, of our nation.

From across our nation,
People quickly came.
Lending, their fellow countrymen, a hand.

From school children to the elderly,
Helping however they can.
To enable others, to feel real grand.

Right across the earth
Amazed at what they've seen
People are asking questions
About, our Lord.

Give us Lord, the words to say
Helping them,
Come to faith in You today

Thank You, Lord
For the protection you gave.
Helping, our countrymen, to be brave.

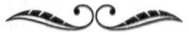

Isaiah 40: 29
   "He gives strength to the weary and increases the power of the weak"

A reflection on the second Christchurch Earthquake and the way every denomination had churches damaged but that did not stop them doing His work and made necessary uniting together to show the much needed love and grace that comes only from The Lord.

Shake Up No.2

Another big shake up
With damage so grand
Death and injury, everywhere How
could this be considered fair?

Lord, from the start
Your hand could already be seen
You already had in place
People to rapidly assist
To help and show Your Love and Grace

Army and navy servicemen on exercise nearby
Many highly skilled doctors right there on the scene
Commencing first aid much quicker
Than one could ever have dreamed.
Many, that don't know You Lord, wondered why.

Disaster relief experts from all over the world
Immediately came to our nation's aid
Joining as one bringing equipment and skills
Helping, our rescue teams.

Christian people showing,
How they love Jesus, their Lord
Following His example
Carrying on His work just as before
Reminding us again,
A church is its' people.

Following their true solid rock,
Jesus, Gods' only son
Not the church buildings
That fail in ground moving shocks.

Was this a call to unite our country, like never before?
Calling all Christians, to wake up and unite
To bring others to know, love and follow You Lord
Overcoming, national damage caused by sin
So, in our country the devil can never win
And for evermore has lost the fight
Then with everyone, following You Lord
Our country and countrymen will be alright.

2 Timothy2 1 Amplified Bible
*   "SO YOU, my son, be strong (strengthened inwardly) in the grace (spiritual blessing) that is (to be found only) in Christ Jesus.*

I wrote this poem after being really blessed with an overflowing calmness and sense of His Grace, during my prayer time the morning after I wrote Part of His Plan. Also on that day I had heard of a situation where a non-Christian was drawn to inquire of a mutual friend what they had that others didn't have as they wanted it.

When On Our Knees

It's at times like these
When we're on our knees
Seeking His face That our Lord
Overfills us with His Grace

Filled and overflowing
His light and love through us are showing

That's when strangers will notice
What we have, saying
"We want what those people have got"

That's exactly how His good news is further spread
When the Bible is not yet being read.

2 Corinthians 3:3
    "Your lives are a letter anyone can read by just looking at you. Christ Himself wrote it—not with ink but with God's living spirit;not chiselled into stone, but carved into human lives - and we publish it."

This poem God inspired me to write over the last 2 days. I was reflecting on how through a very recent & difficult life storm my Lord and Saviour cared for me through. He did this so well that it felt like I was floating on the breeze.
Thank You Lord.

While sailing though Life

While, sailing through life
We come across strife
But we do not sink,
When of Jesus we think.
Slowly and steadily
Right on
Through life's storms we sail
Troubles, worries and strife
Begin to pale.

Join with me then,
Loving, serving and following Him
Accept, His love and peace.
Receive total forgiveness
For all of your sins

Thank You Lord Jesus
For giving Your Life
So we can all have
The best Saviour, teacher and friend
Right through our lives.

Mathew 14:24-27 (The Message)

'Meanwhile, the boat was far out to sea when the wind came up against them and they were battered by the waves. At about four o'clock in the morning, Jesus came toward them walking on the water. They were scared out of their wits. "A ghost!" they said, crying out in terror.

But Jesus was quick to comfort them. "Courage, it's me. Don't be afraid."'

The reassurance that God is in control no matter how stormy life is right now was the inspiration behind this poem

Early One Morn

Awoken early one morn
Way before dawn
Out of the window I peeped

The full moon sharing it's light
Broke the darkness on this gusty night
Clouds of all types and magnitudes being
pushed along at such a rate
It was like they were late... for a very important date

At times one could have despaired
That the moon had totally disappeared
The thing that stood out without any doubt
Was the moon never went away
It was just briefly hidden from sight
At times during that stormy night.

In awe of God's creation that morn
I lay watching those clouds fly by... God spoke to me
Reminding me that even when
My path seems not to be lit with His
light He never goes away!

No matter how dark and grey
The path may be
He is always there shining His light
He never disappears as
He will always love and care for me.

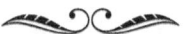

Hebrews 13:5(CEB)

5 *Your way of life should be free from the love of money, and you should be content with what you have. After all, he has said, I will never leave you or abandon you.[a]*

This poem speaks about a night of worship and praise at our church during which a live worship album was recorded.

That Special Night

Heavenly Father,
On that special night,
People came from here and there
To be, all at once in the one same place
In worship praise and prayer.

Before the night had even begun
Your Holy Spirit had already come
The Spirits presence was so strong
It was felt by everyone
Who'd gathered together as one
To worship and praise Your Son

Father, that special night,
Gifts You had given were clearly in sight
Such musical talent ensuring the album would definitely
Be far more than just alright.

So many had gathered together as one
To praise and worship Jesus Your only Son
A mighty album of praise was raised
A new ministry has just begun.

Praise and worship so sincere
The words of praise so clearly sung
That far from the church,
Out in the crystal clear night air,
Loud and clear they hung
Banishing, right then and there,
Satan's, evil spirit of fear,
Totally, from that areas atmosphere.

Father, thank you
For gifting people here
Musical gifts, so obviously clear
That they can lead Your people so beautifully
In worship, praise and prayer.

2 Samuel 22:50 (CEB)
   ***50** "That's why I thank you, Lord, in the presence of the nations. That's why I sing praises to your name."*

The inspiration for the poem below came one wet day as I sat watching some TV. I became horrified that over eight weeks before Christmas the advertisements were already putting pressure on people to spend up large on material gifts with not one mention of the real reason why we celebrate Christmas.

Christmas Thoughts

Christmas time will soon be here
It hardly seems like it has been a year
Since, we thanked God for sending Jesus down here.

That wondrous Star
Seen by all from near and far,
Signals Lord Jesus birth.
Sent, in love… from God above,
To all folk here on Earth.

That wondrous star, sent from above
Signals our Saviours birth
The love He brings should make people sing
And fill their homes with mirth.
BUT

As Christmas time again rolls around
Peace, love and joy;
should in every home abound
Sadly in many homes,
Only stress and tension are found.
It seems so unfair that everywhere,
We are pressured to buy so much gear
Much more than many can afford.

So this year my fellow Christians
let's remember the true reason for the season.
Showing God's love and peace for evermore.
By bringing to the doors of the poor
The Good news from our Heavenly Father up above.

This poem is an appreciation of the greatest gift of all time.

The Precious Gift

Lord Jesus
You were born in a cave
To Earthly parents who were so so brave.
At a time on Earth when things were so grave.

Your Father Our Heavenly dad
Sent You A tiny wee babe
So in years to come
You Lord, His only son
Could give Your life as the ultimate sacrifice

Lord,
You are that precious gift
You made that ultimate sacrifice
When you died on the cross at Calvary
Taking our sins upon yourself
From all our sins You set us eternally free

May we all, forever remember
The real reason why we celebrate your birth
Spreading the Good news ; unto the ends of the Earth.

Peter 1:3
Praise be to the God and Father of our Lord Jesus Christ! In his great mercy he has given us new birth into a living hope through the resurrection of Jesus Christ from the dead,

I was wondering how to word my new year's greeting to my friends. Immediately this poem arrived in my mind. Inspired by recognition of how much alike the start of a new year is to the new start Christ gave us when we gave our lives to Him.

New Year's Eve

It's new years' eve.
Time to reflect
What the years been like
Was it one we would rather forget
Or one to celebrate with joy.

The start of a new year
A chance to remember
Jesus sacrificed His life
So we could start fresh new lives

So as tomorrows dawn
Brings a brand new year
Instead of holding back
For fear of Spiritual attack.

Now is the time for us all
To engage another gear
Demonstrating
Gods' Love and Care
To all folk everywhere.

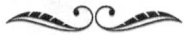

Corinthians 5:17 (CEB)
    So then, if anyone is in Christ, that person is part of the new creation. The old things have gone away, and look, new things have arrived!

This one God gave me the words to when I was helping with car parking for a funeral of a longstanding member of our church. God had me reflecting on those newer Christians and was wanting me to encourage them to plunge themselves into His everlasting arms at these times.

At Times of Loss

At times of loss when feeling sad,
We must remember,
We have an awesome Heavenly Dad.

He knows,. just how we feel
He sent, Jesus to The Cross.
To ensure a home up above,
For all who accept His Love,
And all the gifts of The Cross

So cling onto His amazing love,
Rest In His comforting embrace.
And soon you will be back
Speeding along life's racetrack
Destination Heaven!

An amazing reunion
Awaits you there… With many
You have always held so dear.

"Come to me, all you who are weary and burdened, and I will give you rest."

Mathew 11:28

*Written after a text letting me know a friends elderly frail dad
was very low. God immediately laid this poem line and word perfect
on my heart while praying for them both within minutes of that text
coming through. Telling me that He would let me know whenever
& wherever He wants it shared*

Your Time to Go

We all know,
It was, your time to go
into Heaven above.

While we're sad,
You had to go
We've released you, with love.

Knowing, you're resting
Deep in,
His, wonderful love.

Those left below
Want you to know
God's unfailing, infinite love
Sent down from Heaven above
Has. us wrapped securely In His unfailing arms
Looking, after us all.

He,
Already has in place
Friends & people, we don't yet know
Providing comfort,
Care and love
For those left here below.

John 3:16
"For God loved the world so much that He gave His one and only Son,
so that everyone who believes in Him will not perish but have eternal life."
(New Living Translation)

At the start of a short prayer retreat God challenged me to turn the following phrase into a form of poetry.

"Rise Up; Reach Out; And Help Bring My People Home"

Relax you can do it
Invest in others
Seek out the lost
Encourage gently with

Unlimited energy
Praising Him continually

Restoring Hope
Enveloped in Love
Anchored in His Family
Coaching gently as you do a child
Helping them to grow

Overcoming Satan
Undoing all Satans damage
Time involved is irrelevant... It's His time not our time

Answer openly their questions
Never give up
Deny Satan any opportunity

Healing in Your time Lord
Enduring our cross for Your sacrifice Lord
Leading the lost to You
Protecting them from worldly values

Boldly step out
Reassure new members
Invest in the faltering
New confidence You give us
Growth for all

Many millions more are
Yet to come home

Preparing them for
Evermore being able to
Overcome
Prayerfully & powerfully, problems… as they learn to
Loyally follow Our Lord Jesus Christ…
and grow to know they'll be
Eternally looked after

Heading steadily
Onward and upward
Majestically homeward bound for
Eternity.

VOLUME 2

Acknowledgements

I would like to acknowledge and thank all those who have encouraged me to publish the poetry God inspires me to write.

I, especially want to acknowledge Pastors Pip Batten, Steve Walsh of City West Church, New Plymouth and Pastor Jon Hales (now at Riverside Christian Fellowship Kaiapoi NZ) for the mentoring they have given me since I have been attending City West Church. They have been a key part of my spiritual growth that lead to the confidence to share my poetry with people I do not know.

To _www.Biblegateway.com_ for having a website that made adding the scripture verses I wanted so easy.

What God has done in my life (updated)

God first looked after me when I was born to loving parents on 9th January 1954.

He ensured even though mum and dad had clashing blood types I only got mild after effects mentioned below. (Many babies were severely disabled or died before birth with the RH negative factor in those days.)

2 ½ years later He gave mum the strength to carry on and do a good job raising my sister and me when dad died 8 months after contracting Polio

He helped me through school especially the early years when I was teased both for a speech impediment and co-ordination problems

He ensured I got speech help at primary school. I hated this as a 7 to 9 year old! As I often would miss out on class swimming time because of speech. Speech consisted of learning many poems and rhyming jingles. As always God knew what He was doing; 50 years in the future He'd use this for His work!

Mum ensured we attended Sunday School and when I was about 13 at a Presbyterian Easter Camp in Eltham, Taranaki I gave my life to Him.

He ensured I was accepted and passed my Community Nursing course and gave me a passion for the elderly and significantly disabled.

In 1985 I fell in love and got married

God upheld, loved and often carried me through the next 17 years.

In early 1986 I became pregnant with our first son and we were really excited.

Late October the specialist told me (when I was alone) at an antenatal appointment that there was a problem with my babies brain. I would probably have to have a Caesarean Section and baby would be 6 weeks premature and may be severely disabled and not live!

The paediatricians had other ideas and my precious son was carried to 38 weeks and while John has some significant disabilities God ensured I did not have a dead baby but a precious loving son.

Praise God for giving the plumber whose own baby had hydrocephalus the skills to design the first shunt to bypass the blockage. Without this dad thousands of babies world-wide would not have lived over the previous 20 years including John!

God carried me supporting me with Christian Music and Poetry while John went through 17 lots of brain surgery in his first 7 years of life Including when John was about 18 months my marriage broke up due mainly to my husband not admitting he wasn't coping with the continued stress of John's medical problems.

When John was about 15 he caught a very bad virus and lost heaps of weight, no doctor thought to check his blood medication levels and one level got far too high this caused him to become extremely violent without warning. God carried me giving me the wisdom to do a very difficult thing for any mother; to place John in care for my own and his 13yr old brothers safety.

In November 2006 I was listening to Life FM in the car one morning before going in to teacher aide the very high needs student I was working with, when I heard the quote *"If God takes you to it He will get you through it"* and thought to myself gee that will be really useful to share one day.

Under 36 hours later I was the one needing that quote to help me through God's timing always perfect!

Contact had always been maintained with John and 2 years later God kept his brother and me safe when John came home for a two hour visit and due to things earlier in the day John lost it putting James and my lives in danger for a short period.

During this period God prompted me to follow John's brother and change churches to attend City West Church where I could worship without well-meaning people asking how John was. Amazing the difference this made and I found a much greater depth to my relationship with my Lord.

God gave me the wisdom to see through my feelings and make the decision that John could never visit again unless accompanied by staff.

That night I cried out to My Lord what am I to do now?

Next morning, I awoke still feeling shattered WHEN... the room suddenly became full of God's peace.

I thought I was ready for what He was going to tell me to do,

BUT I CERTAINLY WAS NOT EXPECTING WHAT HE SAID TO ME!!

As soon as I was soaking up His peace God said to me

"You are to sell this place and move out to live with and care for your mother, for me" I replied asking him "what was that last part, Lord?" He replied "you heard me, you can do it, act quickly. You are to move by the start of the school year" Several friends and extended family told me: "it won't work," "you can't do it" **BUT** For the first time in my life I knew emphatically the devil was trying to derail my life and God's plan.

Ignoring all the comments I obeyed God. The house sold quickly before it was put on the market; for the required amount God's confirmation to me. To say the next few months were trying is a major understatement. But with God's helping hand, we made it through.

Women's conference 08: God gave me 3 messages. Go through the waters of baptism, tell your story, I am all and more than you need.

My water baptism in July 08 Again the devil tried to derail this. I woke with an asthma attack that day which should have seen me in A & E not at church. No way was I missing my baptism, using heaps of ventolin to get there. God's awesome response HE removed troublesome asthma from my life that night.

Only a few months later I was baptised in the Holy Spirit and God turned up massively the speed on the escalator of growth in my Christian faith. Within weeks a Christian friend who didn't know about it asked me what had changed. She said. "You have so much confidence, you are sharing openly what has changed?"

God really ignited a passion to get Christian Poetry recorded and out there on CD at this stage and a few weeks later a friend challenged me to write some of my own. The very next day God gave me the words to my first poem. In the last two years God has:

- Healed 25yr old injuries to my neck and shoulder ligaments.
- Prompted me to get over my technophobia and start using technology to share the poetry he inspires me to write. *www.life-poetry-to-encourage.com* is a direct result of obedience to this instruction.
- He continues to challenge, stretch and look after me. Enabling me to bless others by sharing His unconditional love for everyone through my poetry

Update since volume 1

Since publishing Volume 1 God has continued to inspire me to write Christian Poetry through messages at church and events in my life.

I was always determined I would never embrace Social Media but My Lord had very different ideas and shortly after I published Volume 1, He used several people telling me they should be on Facebook to remove my determination against Facebook etc. Since I have started posting on Facebook, I have realized that He needed me to encourage many people who otherwise my poems would not have helped.

It is very humbling when you are contacted and thanked by someone overseas within a few minutes of posting a poem on Facebook saying that by posting it I had saved their life.

To this day I still cannot write poetry on any other subject.

I am only My Lords' pen.

I never know when, where or the reason why He wants a poem written and published in a specific place and at a specific time.

God is waiting and wanting to look after you!

He has always loved you!

He will in turn use you to spread His good word.

May all who read the poems in this second volume be blessed mightily.

God Bless
Janice Mannex

Woke one morning thinking how life so far would have been almost impossible if I had not known Jesus Christ as my Lord and Saviour.

Down in the Dumps? Good News My Friend

Feeling down in the dumps?
Think there's no way out?
Your life
DOES NOT NEED to end.!!!
Your life
DOES NOT HAVE to end.!!!

My friend, I have
such good news.
I have
the ultimate friend
He is
a friend to all!
He's just
waiting for your
Please Help me call.!!

His name is
Jesus
He is
God's only son
He loves everyone

Jesus wants
your life's
battle to be won.

Jesus loves
And
cares for you
He always will.

Take hold
of His hand
And you will land
On your feet,
They will be
tapping out
A happy beat

You then will be
Running back
up the hill
Your Saviour
to meet
With a smile
on your dial
Instead
of a frown.

Now
don't go thinking
You've sunk
too far down

There's a ladder
Right down
from Heaven

It extends
Right down
to your feet.

Jesus will
help you
That ladder
to climb

Never leaving
your side
He is
the ultimate guide.

©JEM 9th June 2013

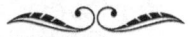

Hebrews 13:5 (Common English Bible)
Your way of life should be free from the love of money, and you should be content with what you have. After all, he has said, I will never leave you or abandon you.

Inspired by a message reminding us that Jesus is ready to listen 24 hours a day 7 days a week.

Jesus, Listener Extraordinaire!

Jesus is our listener
He answers prayers…
We're unable to share

He listens…
to all our requests
And clearly hears…
our hearts
most secret fears.

He knows
all our needs
before we ask
Removes
all our worries
and cares.

Jesus Christ
You
Love us
unconditionally
Inspire us
to reach
out to others

Seek out
the lost
Teach us
to be more
like You

You
Endured The Cross
Never let us down
Eternally care
Rescue and restore us.

Jesus
You are our
Listener
extraordinaire!!!
Thank You Lord.

©JEM 1st June 2013

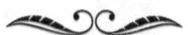

Matthew 7:7 (CEB)
7 "Ask, and you will receive. Search, and you will find. Knock, and the door will be opened to you.

A reflection on difficult times when John was young; how I managed to overcome with the help of My Lord and Saviour

How Did You Cope?

How do you cope?
Was often heard
No point in not
I would reply

It'll only be worse
if I don't try
They'd often reply
that's just absurd

You see I'd say
I have a
very special friend
Who will
always help me

No matter
how often
No matter
how long
No matter
the time of day

He's always
there for me
Especially
when things
Seem to
go wrong.

Their eyes
would light up
Their ears
turned on

Minds trying
to work out
Who Just who
Was this man
I knew.

Who was
so good
He could
get me through?

Where does
he live?
Where does
he work?

So he can
just stop work
And to your aid
always come

Folk
His name is
Jesus
He is
God's only son
He'll help
anyone to overcome

I know
this for sure
He's done
it for me

Just come to Him
on bended knee
And humbly ask
Him into your life

You too then
will be able
to cope better
than ever before

With Jesus
on board
our perfect coach!

Jesus is
our ultimate friend
For Him
our friendship
never ends!

©JEM 9th July 2014

1 Chronicles 29:12 (CEB)

You are the source of wealth and honour and You rule over all In Your hand are strength and might and it is in Your power To magnify and strengthen all

This poem was inspired by a message at church on the special hope we have through Jesus Christ.

Hope That Lasts

People's hope
is based
In many things.

For many people
Their foundation
for hope is not
always the best.

Hope in
work place success
Even when
they do their best.

They may not
pass that test
Leaving them
a total mess.

Hope based
in material things
Of insecurity rings

Material things
can disappear
Into seemingly
thin air

Creating,
much hurt
and despair.

Hope based in others
May seem fine
Some of them however
let others down
Causing that hope
to start to drown

Hope in
Jesus Christ
however
Will forever be
your strong tower

Hope in Him
Will never founder
He'll be your rock
Forever more
He's theonly
real safe ground.

Eternal hope
Is only found
In Jesus Christ
where it abounds.

©JEM 4am 11 /11/2013

Psalm 33:20 (CEB)
We put our hope in the Lord. He is our help and our shield

This poem is dedicated to all who lost loved ones and those who were badly injured in the Oklahoma Tornado, and any other tragedies that have occurred since.

Just A Note To Say

Just a note to say
I'm thinking
and praying
for you today
with the tragedy
that's come your way

When things
like this happen
It's hard for us
to fathom out
How today
this can be
Part of God's plan
in any way!

But into this
Turmoil and tragedy
God's love
will flow,
Through those
helping out
here below.

Many more people,
Will Our Lord
and Saviour know
Through the many
He had ready,
To race
to that place.

To show
His love,
His care
and His grace
So they could
flood that place
With everything
needed on that day.

POEM © JEM21/5/2013

Jeremiah 30:17 (NRSV)
   "For I will restore health to you, and your wounds I will heal, says the Lord,"

Inspired through a message at a women's conference in Hawera New Zealand.

Come Sit In His Shade

Come Sit in His Shade
Be still and receive
For Jesus Christ
God's only son
Wants to lead you.

Wants to bless
You so richly today!
Yes You!
Right here and now!

Don't go telling me
You are not good enough.
Jesus loves,
Jesus forgives everyone!

His love is so pure
It will always
Forgive,
Free and
Restore
From all... Yes all
That's gone before!

So come now
Sit in His shade
Rest and be blessed
And
You will find you are
No longer stressed!

Rested and refreshed
You will be able
To help those others
Desperately needing
To be less stressed

Ask them to join you
So they can be blessed
Having sat in His shade
They too will
No longer being stressed!

@JEM 5am 30 March 2014

Mathew 11:28(The Message)
    Are you tired? Worn out? Burned out on religion? Come to me. Get
away with me and you'll recover your life.
    I'll show you how to take a real rest.

This poem was inspired by God after I prayed asking for the words to help friends who had been wayward when younger and were convinced that they had been too bad for God to love them.

Life's Like That

Life's like that
That's a fact
Jesus loves you
So is that.

We've all
gone wrong
As life
has gone on
Jesus helps us
To get along.

We've all sinned
So
where to begin
Jesus forgives us
Welcoming us in

Jesus meets us
where we are at
No tests to pass
That's a fact

No standards to meet
Jesus always
Takes us back
Standing us strongly
Back on our feet

How to get on
His life bus
Jesus teaches us
As we go along
Till to Him
We sing a song.

Now go tell
All you meet
At work
At home
Or
Down the street

Doing so
Until the day
His life bus
Takes us all the way
To Heaven above
To celebrate with Him

©JEM 20

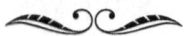

Psalm 103: 3-5 (The Message)

He forgives your sins—every one. He heals your diseases—every one. He redeems you from hell—saves your life! He crowns you with love and mercy—a paradise crown. He wraps you in goodness— beauty eternal. He renews your youth—you're always young in his presence.

A reflection on how yet again My Lord kept me safe when life was a bit rough!

Jesus Our LifeJacket

When life's tide starts
Giving you
a rough ride.
Put on
your life jacket
Ask Jesus alongside

Jesus is our lifejacket
A perfect fit
in every storm

Whether that storm's
big or small
He'll get you through
that rough patch
No trouble at all.

When life's again
upon
an ultra-smooth highway
Jesus will
always be alongside
Instantly ready
to deploy
and catch you
next time you hit
a rough patch.

So don't forget to
talk to Him often
He will
smooth out
Those, bumpy
country lanes
And ensure
life's road
Is not too
much of a pain!

© JEM 25th May 2013

Hebrews 13:5 The Message (MSG)
Don't be obsessed with getting more material things. Be relaxed with what you have.
Since God assured us, "I'll never let you down, never walk off and leave you,"

Just woke one morning with this poem in my mind already complete.

Our Shepherd

Jesus Christ
You are my Saviour :
You saved me
from my sins

Help me,
to show others
Just how easy
It is to begin
A life with You
free from sin.

Jesus Christ
You are my healer :
Thank you
for healing me

Help me
to tell others
All about Thee

Jesus Christ
You are
my encourager
You've encouraged me
out of timidity

So I can
openly share
what
You have
done for me

Jesus Christ
You are
our protector
You erect a
hedge of protection
all around us

So NO harm
can come
to those
Who choose
to jump aboard
"The Life with You"
work bus

Jesus Christ
You are my helper
When we need
a helping hand

You are so
steadfastly reliable
Sending down
from Heaven above
A helping hand

so big
Accompanied
with heaps of love
Enabling me
to help Your land

Jesus Christ
You are
my enricher
You add
Heaps of richness
to my life

Help me to
show the riches
You add
To those
whose lives
to them
Seem hopeless
and so bad.

Jesus Christ
You are my restorer…
You restore lives
Worldwide everyday

May I help others
To come to know
The restoration
that comes

When they
Come to You
And
Do life Your way

Jesus Christ
You are my Defender
You are the
only defender I need

You provide
The ultimate armour
The ultimate defence
Of this I am
very sure indeed!

Saviour,
Healer,
Encourager,
Protector,
Enricher,
Restorer
Defender
What a special Shepherd
we're blessed with!

Lord Jesus Christ,
Forever
I will thank You
Forever
I will praise You,

From the bottom
of my heart
For being
OUR
ultimate guiding Shepherd.

©JEM 4th June 2013

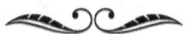

Psalm 23:4 The Message
   Even when the way goes through Death Valley, I'm not afraid when you walk at my side.
   Your trusty shepherd's crook makes me feel secure.

Woke one Sunday morning reflecting on how many different seasons God had lead me safely through. The evening service message God used to show me to be careful not to get stuck but to be ready to open and move into the next folder.

Our Lives are Like a Pile of Folders

Our lives
Are like a
pile of folders
All stacked ready
for us to action.

Each folder taking
Some time to complete
Challenges abound
Deadlines;
we just have to meet!

The next one waiting
Ready to be taken
from its holder
Inside this folder
He has put
New tasks for us
to complete

Our Lord
has designed them…
To make us bolder
He will keep us
steady and strong
So we can steer others
Away from all wrong

Guiding
all those we meet
Through our actions
Back to the correct street

Until it's time
for us to greet
Our Lord and Saviour
Kneeling at his feet
Our lifes' folders
Now all complete.

©JEM 4am 4/8/2013

"Ecclesiastes 3 CEB
    There's a season for everything and a time for every matter under the
heavens: a time for giving birth and a time for dying, a time for planting
and a time for uprooting what was planted, a time for killing and a time
for healing, a time for tearing down and a time for building up, . . ."

Inspired, by a message at church urging us to make sure we were giving God our best effort for His kingdom.

All In for Him?

All in for Him?
All in for your team?
Sounds like
a good scheme to me.

Jesus is
All in for us
How about joining
His life bus?

Lifelong is the trip
So you'd better
get a good grip.

The road at times
Will be rough
Jesus will help
You to betough

Resting on Him
Is a must
And in Him
Totally placing
your trust.

Although the going
may be slow
Jesus your hand
won't let go.

When you're injured
Or you're down
Jesus doesn't
greet you
With a frown
He will never ever
Let you down

Jesus has
for you
A part to play
How about
asking Him
What that
is today?

It could be
About things
you think
Would be
NO WAY!

There's a place
in Jesus heart
A special position
in His Team

He has already
set it apart
It's just waiting
For you to
join the team

You can
jump aboard
From where
you're at
No tests or
trials to pass
That's a fact
All you
have to do
is ask.

Your life
in a spin
Jesus welcomes
Everyone
So why not join in ?

Become all in
GIVE
your life to Him,

God's Only Son
A better life for you
Will certainly begin.

©JEM 29 August 2013

Mathew 4:18-20 NIV 18

As Jesus was walking beside the Sea of Galilee, he saw two brothers, Simon called Peter and his brother Andrew. They were casting a net into the lake, for they were fishermen. 19 "Come, follow me," Jesus said, "and I will send you out to fish for people." 20 At once they left their nets and followed him

Inspired through a message when visiting a church in Dunedin New Zealand

Because

Because can be taken
In many ways
It can improve
Or destroy
someone's day.

Bible tells us
Embrace His grace
Completely trust it
Anchor our lives on Him
Unfailing Love
Saviour of all
Eternally available

Because He lives
Embrace His Grace
Call on His name
Always honour Him
Unfailing Love
Saviour of all
Eternally available

Because He died
Everyone has hope
Completely forgiven

Awesome gift
Unending Peace
Son of God
Everlasting Encourager

Believe in Christ
Encourage others
Complete trust is a must
Allow Christ too
Unconditionally forgive you
Saved by His Grace
Encourage others

Now because of this
Don't be amiss

Best spread the news
Everywhere on Earth
Come to Our Lord
Accept His forgiveness
Unlimited is His love
Saved by His grace
Eternally blessed.

© JEM 17-11-13

Proverbs 3:5-6 (NIV)
Trust in the Lord with all your heart and lean not on your own understanding; in all your ways submit to him, and he will make your paths straight

Upon waking I was thanking God for the sacrifice the ANZAC soldiers made when they gave their lives so we could live in freedom. When the words to this poem immediately came to mind so vividly that I just had to pen the poem

Sunrise Sunset

The beauty
of the sunrise
The glorious sunset
Just parts of
God's Creation
Let's be sure that…
This we
do not forget.

At each sunset
Let's remember
the sunset
Jesus met
on Good Friday
So He could arise
On Easter Sunday

When we
give our lives
to serve our God
We meet
our first sunset
Our old lives
getting left behind
at that sunset

We arise
completely washed clean
At that moment
A beautiful new life
in us does arise
Like the
beautiful morning sunrise.

Jesus's ultimate sacrifice
Let 's not forget
Thanking Him for it
Each and every
glorious sunset

Each sunrise
then let us bring
Praise and worship…
Heartily singing
thanks to our God, Our King.

©JEM 26th April 2013

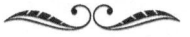

Jerimiah 31:35 (Good News Translation)
    The Lord provides the sun for light by day, the moon and the stars
to shine at night.
    He stirs up the sea and makes it roar; his name is the Lord Almighty

This poems' first two verses were already on my heart when I woke very early in the morning the rest followed as soon as I started typing.

Heavenly Father

Our Heavenly Father
When like sheep
we go astray
Gently says
come on home
I'll show you
the best way.

Heavenly Father
You'll never
say to me
Not again
Ask me
again another day
I have
no more time for thee.

Heavenly Father
You sent
Jesus your Son
He died for me
On Calvary's Tree
To, completely
set me free.

Heavenly Father
Thank You
You cared enough
To send Your Son
Completely forgiving me
So I'm eternally set free.

©JEM 1st December 2013

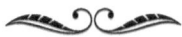

Luke 15:8-10 The Message Bible

"Or imagine a woman who has ten coins and loses one. Won't she light a lamp and scour the house, looking in every nook and cranny until she finds it? And when she finds it you can be sure she'll call her friends and neighbours: 'Celebrate with me! I found my lost coin!' Count on it—that's the kind of party God's angels throw every time one lost soul turns to God."

Inspired by a discussion at a church home group on 5th March 2014

Building Bridges is a Must

Building bridges
is a must
Reaching out first
The way to grow

Investing time
So each other
we know

Defining
the pathways
Along which
we will go

God sent us;
The only bridge
back to Him

His Son
Jesus Christ
Essential,
expensive and eternal;

But Oh so so
Worth the cost.

Supporting structures
Need to stay strong;

Build bridges to Jesus
So you
don't go wrong.

Burning bridges
tear apart
Friendships bedded
Deep down
in the heart.

Sometimes
mending
Burnt bridges
Is a must
Trusting Jesus
Then is a must

No better
bridge mender
Will you find
Than Our Lord
Jesus Christ.
No matter how long
You search your mind

©JEM 6am 16th March 2014

John 13:34-35 the Message
*"Let me give you a new command: Love one another. In the same way
I loved you, you love one another. This is how everyone will recognize that
you are my disciples—when they see the love you have for each other."*

Inspired by the message spoken that Sunday night at church.

Climb That Sycamore Tree

Step out in faith
Climb that Sycamore tree
Position yourself
So Jesus you'll see.

You
Jesus will
definitely see
And He'll call
you down

To meet
in the street
Then to
your place
You both
will retreat.

Jesus knows
You come
on bended knee
Confident and ready
for tasks
He has for
you to complete.

Even when
tasks here below
Are In places
you sure
don't want to go.

© JEM 9.45 pm 30/1/2014

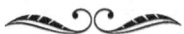

Luke 19:9-10 The Message
    Jesus said, "Today is salvation day in this home! Here he is: Zacchaeus, son of Abraham!
    For the Son of Man came to find and restore the lost."

This poem came out of the sudden loss of a valued member of our church home group as a result of an accident while serving Our Lord. The reassurances My Lord gave me as I asked Him Why?

Initially a tribute I was not going to publish it but have been prompted to do so by My Lord. I pray it will give all those who read it strength at times of sudden loss.

We Don't Understand

Lord,
Yet again
Your timing
we don't understand
But rest
we must knowing
You had
everything planned

Every precise detail
You knew
Needed to play
Its' own special part
In Your master plan.

Lord we give
You thanks
We know
Your son,
our friend
Is now home
with You

Struggles to
keep on
keeping on
For You Lord
Now are over
and
You have said
Welcome home,
Good and faithful servant.

© JEM 2013

Proverbs 3:6 (The Message Bible)
Trust God from the bottom of your heart; don't try to figure out everything on your own.

Inspired when reflecting on the blessings that God provided even when the initial answer to prayer was presenting problems.

An Answer to Prayer

An answer to prayer,
Appeared to be near
A special present
was now here.

New computer systems to learn
Not all going right
I soon was beginning
to despair that night

Into my ear came
a still quiet voice
"Be aware!!

Don't despair
I am right here
Satan is trying
to put you
Into a spirit of fear"

Satan thought
Here is my
chance to attack
I am glad to say
I heard that still
quiet voice that day

Next thing I knew
The phone did ring
News of an
unexpected visit
That call did bring.

A new manager
was bringing
My special son
to see me
John wanted
To show me
his new technology
So I could share
In some
of his glee.

That new person
Just happened to be
Highly qualified in
Computer technology

He took a look
Then said to me
Something is wrong...
I'll fix it for you
Don't open that whatever you do!

John's manager
Gave me
a gift that day

A protection program
And
an awesome visit from John

I'm so glad for the
still quiet voice that day
And that
I listened to the
still quiet voice that day.
For the complete
answer to prayer
was indeed very near.

©JEM 4th January 2014

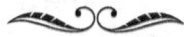

Acts 16:25 & 26 (CEB)
   Around midnight Paul and Silas were praying and singing hymns to God, and the other prisoners were listening to them. 26 All at once there was such a violent earthquake that it shook the prison's foundations. The doors flew open and everyone's chains came loose.

Inspired through a message about how blessed we are to have a Heavenly Father and that the very early Christians obeyed God.

I Thank You

Thank You
Heavenly Father
For sending your Son
I am so glad
He did come.
Down to Earth
To show us all
How to live life
close to you.

Thank You
Heavenly Father
Mary and Joseph,
chose to obey
Not running away in fright
At the task
You gave them that day.

Thank You Lord
You obeyed Your Father
Even when it meant
Dying on Calvary's Tree
Rising again
to set me free.

Thank You Lord
Your disciples
took the time
To record
Your words,
Your actions.

The Bible now
centuries later
teaches us
How to
be more like You.

Lord
Help me
to always be
Ready,
willing to obey
So I can
inspire others at
the appointed time

©JEM 9pm 29th December 2013

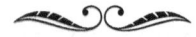

A reflection on the many times My Lord Jesus Christ has been there and carried me through these times.

In Times of Sadness Times of Pain

In times of sadness,
times of pain
In times of sickness,
times of rain
Turn to Jesus
the ultimate friend

My friend,
you may
not comprehend
How Jesus
can be such a friend

Be encouraged
do not despair
Jesus waits
for your prayer.

Give
your heart to Jesus
That's all it takes
my friend
For these circumstances

to start coming
to an end.

Do not think…
your life's too stink
You've done
too many bad things
Jesus will forgive you
He is the forgiveness king!

So reach out
To Jesus the friend
who always cares
He's always
waiting for someone new

To come to Him in prayer
He will
break through your pain
You will
have happiness again.

©JEM May 26th 2013

Jeremiah 32:40 (Common English Bible)
    40 I will make an everlasting covenant with them, never to stop
treating them graciously. I will put into their hearts a sense of awe for me
so that they won't turn away from me.

A reflection on a message reminding us that we all have special jobs to do and that no two are the same.

A Job I've Got For You

A job
I've got for you today
Do not delay
You need
To start it right away!

Don't let life's storms
Put you off course
I need you to stay
Right with this job
All the way
Not just today.

Speak and sing
Of Jesus our king
Again and again
So in all people's ears
His name does ring.

Speak and Sing
Of His total care
Do it everywhere
At home at work
And in the air.

Speak and sing
Again and again
Of His perfect love
After all it is
Everyone's perfect
Safety glove!

It's totally free
No matter the task
Let them know
All they have to do is ask.

Speak and sing
Of Jesus ourking.
The love peace and joy
That knowing Himbrings.

©JEM 4am 22 June 2013

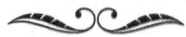

1 Corinthians 12:27-31 The Message Bible
   You are Christ's body—that's who you are! You must never forget this. Only as you accept your part of that body does your "part" mean anything. You're familiar with some of the parts that God has formed in his church, which is his "body": Apostles, prophets, teachers, miracle workers, healers, helpers, organizers, those who pray in tongues. But it's obvious by now, isn't it, that Christ's church is a complete Body and not a gigantic, unidimensional Part? It's not all Apostle, not all Prophet, not all Miracle Worker, not all Healer, not all Prayer in Tongues, not all Interpreter of Tongues. And yet some of you keep competing for so-called "important" parts.

Inspired by a message reminding us Jesus is already up in the throne room of Heaven awaiting us.

Heaven's Throne Room

Heaven's throne room
Already occupied
No little spaces
In which Satan can hide.

Our Heavenly Father
rules supreme.
Jesus Christ sits
right alongside
Better than any dream.

Lord Jesus
we thank you
For setting us free
When, you died for us
On Calvary's tree.
Our sins
forever forgiven.

Our sins
banished forever
To the slippery slide
Satan finds himself on
When in our lives
he tries to find
A very sneaky
place to hide.

The veil pushed aside
We're forgiven and free
Able to join You there
And Lord
we are able
To sit on Your Knee.!

On guard forever
we must be
Drawing ever closer
Lord to Thee
Satan's attempts then
Will go for a slide

As there will be no place
For him to hide
And ultra-alert
To any attempt we'll be

©JEM 23rd August 2013

Luke 22:69 (GNT)
69 But from now on the Son of Man will be seated at the right side of Almighty God."

This poem is inspired by a massive challenge God laid in front of me. Recently in a seemingly busy few weeks God challenged me to compile and publish a book of all the poems He had inspired me to write at that point. Then He laid in my heart the time frame He wanted it completed by less than 3 weeks. With finance and a publishing firm also to find I obeyed and He has blessed me massively.

His Time Makes Room

Sometimes Our Lord
sets us tasks to do
in a very short time

We may think
It's far too big a task
I can't make that!

How will
I get this done
let alone that!

That date
will be here
far toosoon!

Remember He's
there to help
His Father created time
In your schedule…
He will make the room

Trust Him give it a go
And on you…
His blessings will flow.

© poem JEM 27th April 2013

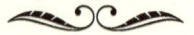

The setting for this poem was my home province had seen some a nasty violent attack in the previous week. This s lead me to praying for people overseas who live their lives in fear and thanking Him that in New Zealand we are so blessed.

Lord... So Often Do We Hear

Lord, so often,
we do hear
Of others living
lives in fear.

Fear of this
or fear of that
Some of their fears
not even fact.

May we
be the ones
To show them that
They can live
day to day
Without that fear
And that's a fact.

Improving
Their lives everyday
Getting alongside them
In, all sorts of ways.

Making them
of You aware
Of Your Love
and Your care
How only You
can take away
All that fear.

Showing them how,
To trust in You
So Lord,
they ask You
To, see them through.

Then to them Lord
You will be the:
Forever Friend
Awesome Anchor
Everlasting Encourager
Rescuing Redeemer.

You are to me
Then they too
Forever will be
Free from fear
Thanks toThee.

© JEM 1-8-2013

Colossians 3:15 (ESV)
*   15 And let the peace of Christ rule in your hearts, to which indeed you were called in one body. And be thankful.*

A reflection on all the pressure commercialization of this special Holy event puts on people many that do not know Our Lord.

Christmas Thoughts

Christmas time
will soon be here
It hardly seems like
it has been a year
Since, we thanked God
For sending
Jesus down here.

That wondrous Star
Seen by all
from near and far,
Signals Lord Jesus birth
Sent in love
from God above,
To all folk
here on Earth.

That wondrous star,
sent from above
Signals
our Saviours birth
The love He brings,

Should make people sing
And fill their homes
with mirth.

As Christmas time
again rolls around
Peace, love and joy;
Should
in every home abound

BUT sadly
in many homes,
Only stress
and tension are found.

It seems so unfair
that everywhere,
We are pressured
to buy
so much gear
Much more than
many can afford.

So this year
my fellow Christians
Let's remember
the true reason
For the season.

BY bringing to
the doors of the poor
God's love and
peace for evermore.
The good news from
Our Heavenly Father up above.

© JEM 2013

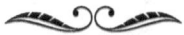

Luke2:11 (NIV)
Today in the town of David a Saviour has been born to you; he is the Messiah, the Lord. 12 This will be a sign to you: You will find a baby wrapped in cloths and lying in a manger."

Just woke one morning and as I opened the curtains the words to this just flowed.

Open the Door & Be Blessed So Much More

Heavenly Father
I thank you
this morning
As I gaze out
upon your dawning sky
Many clouds are drifting by.

Some near
Some far
Some in between

Some dark
Some gloomy
Some clear
Some bright

Reminding me
Our walk through life
Sometimes
has to
Involve strife.

With
Your Only Son
Jesus Christ
in our lives
We are assured
it will always end up right.

When we are struggling
He will assist us
Removing the burden
When it is too much.

At the right time
He provides
Joy for the sad
Strength for the weak
Energy for the tired
Supplies for the needy
And so so much more

How can I
be so sure?
He has done
that for me
since I opened
my hearts door
and asked Him in.

So if you haven't yet
Asked Jesus in
What are you
still waiting for?

Go on
Answer His knocks
UNLOCK your hearts door
He so wants to come in
And bless you
so much more.

© JEM 13/4/2014.

Romans 5:10 GNT
We were God's enemies, but he made us his friends through the death of his Son. Now that we are God's friends, how much more will we be saved by Christ's life!

This was inspired reflecting on what my Lord and Saviour has done for me and longs to do for so many more.

Now Please Come and Meet

Now please
come and meet
Life's best friend
He's in all
The world's houses
He's on all
the World's streets

He's Jesus Christ
God's only son
My Heavenly Dad
I'm so glad
You sent Him
Thank You

Now Please
Don't tell me
you're too shy
No- one's even willing
To give you a try

Jesus is
With Him You'll be
Bold and outgoing
How do I know
He did that for me.

Now Please
don't tell me
you're too tired.

He'll fill you with
Energy to burn
So about Him
Others can learn.

Now please
don't tell me
you're too poor.

Jesus will pour
provisions from Heaven
through your door

Now please
Don't go thinking
You've been
far too bad.

Jesus will forgive you
Opening the pathway
To your Heavenly Dad

You see
He died
On the Cross at Calvary
For You,
yes I said
You and me!

Setting us free
Eternally
from all bad
we ever had.

For all those
Who with me
love and follow Him

Now please
Don't get stuck
In a place of grief.

Jesus will take you
To a place of peace.

Now please
Don't go thinking
This is impossibly good.

It is only
But a glimpse
of the Jesus I know.

Come to Him now
On bended knee
He'll welcome you in
With so much glee.

And from now on
His amazing love
To you He'll show.

©JEM 15th April 2014 (5.30 am)

John 14:6-7 (The Message Bible)
6-7 Jesus said, "I am the Road, also the Truth, also the Life. No one gets to the Father apart from me. If you really knew me, you would know my Father as well. From now on, you do know him. You've even seen him!"

A poem of thanks.

My Heart is Filled

Lord Jesus
My heart is filled
With thankful glee
As I remember
Your' supreme
love for me.

Such was
Your love for me
You hung
On that cross
At Calvary.

Day one
Day two
Went by
People cried
Why why why.

Day three
You arose!
Yippee Yippee Yippee!
All those
Who love you Lord
Now always will be
Eternally free.

My Heart is filled
with thankful glee
Whenever
I remember
What You do for me.

When I'm weak
You make me strong
Then I can for You
Carry on.

When I'm sad
You make me glad
So I can help others
Not to feel so bad.

When I'm a bit lost
You take my hand
Leading me back
No matter the cost!

When running on empty
You overfill
My fuel tank
So onwards for You
I can still go.

MY heart is filled
With thankful glee
As I remember
Your' supreme
love for me.

©JEM 23/04/2014

John 10:10 (The Message Bible)
A thief is only there to steal and kill and destroy. I came so they can have real and eternal life, more and better life than they ever dreamed.

Fan the flame was inspired by a message encouraging us not to hinder Our Lord's work by not activating gifting's He has given us.

Fan the Flame

Welcome
The Holy Spirit in
Don't hold back
So He can set on fire
Gifts He's placed
deep within.

Fan those flames
Dig deep down
Put on a smile
Instead of a frown

Fan the flames
Activating your gift
Oh Don't delay

This very day
It may rescue
Some folk from strife
And save another's life.

©JEM 6am 25th April 2014

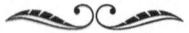

1 Peter 2:4-10 (CEB)

4 Now you are coming to him as to a living stone. Even though this stone was rejected by humans, from God's perspective it is chosen, valuable. 5 You yourselves are being built like living stones into a spiritual temple. You are being made into a holy priesthood to offer up spiritual sacrifices that are acceptable to God through Jesus Christ. 6 Thus it is written in scripture, Look! I am laying a cornerstone in Zion, chosen, valuable. The person who believes in him will never be shamed. [a] 7 So God honours you who believe.

A prayer written during a particularly tough few days.

Lord Please Help

In the midst of trials
Even those
lasting a long while
Lord I pray
Please help me
Not to stray
From Your
narrow pathway.

When problems are rife
Causing much strife
In my life
Lord I pray
Please help me
To still be able
see the way

Shine your light
Clear and bright
So Satan can not
Cause me to get lost

Lord I pray
Help me to dispatch
Sadness that
at times surrounds

For it can
Never ever match
Your Love that abounds

Since you died
For everyone
On Calvary's tree
So we can all
Who love You
be totally free.

© JEM 15 May 2014

Matthew 5:16 *(CEB)*
   In the same way, let your light shine before people, so they can see the good things you do and praise your Father who is in heaven.

Reflecting on how easy it is to forget the people who live close to us may not know Our Lord Jesus Christ

Don't Ignore the People Next Door

Don't Ignore
The people next door
Or maybe further
down your street

That maybe
just where Jesus
wants you to go

Is He
saying to you?
Go there and meet them
They need to know me
NOW MUCH MORE
THAN EVER BEFORE!

It's so
easy to think
The scripture means
We all need to go
To far away countries

So people there
get to know
of Jesus Christ
and His love
to them show.

When just next door
or down the street
The people
you have never met
Need to know
About Jesus Christ
MORE THAN EVER BEFORE

Our Lord
Needing you
to go to their door
Your mission field
could be
right next door!

©JEM 5am 18th June 2014

Mark 5:19 NRSV
    But Jesus refused, and said to him, "Go home to your friends, and tell them how much the Lord has done for you, and what mercy he has shown you."

I was in my quiet time praying I would get what skills my Lord wanted me to pick up from a one day ENGAGE conference that showed folk how to start conversations about spiritual subjects with people we don't really know

Jesus Christ So Badly Wants Them To Know

You so badly
want to reach
The many who
don't yet
have a clue
Who You are

Jesus Christ
You so badly
Want all of them
To know
You have
their name
on Your list

Jesus Christ
You so badly
Want them
to know
The love
You have

for each
and every
one of them

Jesus Christ
You so badly
Want them
to know
total forgiveness
available to them
through You

Jesus Christ
You
so badly
Want them
to know
they can not
have been born
too poor

Jesus Christ
You so badly
Want them
to know
they can not
have been
too bad

Jesus Christ
You so badly

Want them
to know
You care
for them all
no matter
how small

THEY THINK
THEY ARE

Jesus Christ
You so badly
want them
to know
How to
start to know
Who you are

Jesus Christ
You so badly
want each and
every one of us
too share about
things You have
done in our lives
So much more

Jesus Christ
You so badly
want us too realize
the gifts that

You to us
have given
that we still
keep hidden

Jesus Christ
You so badly
want us to realize
there are people
just down the street
in our community
who are yet to get
to know about You

Jesus Christ
Please help us
From now on
To reach out
for You
To the people
who still don't
have a clue
anything at all
about You

Jesus Christ
Thank You
You enable us
To reach out
To step up to
the starting plate

removing
our weaknesses
so we can do
this for You
before it is too late.

When we feel
worthless and useless
You make us
Worthy and Useful

When we feel
Timid and shy
You make us
Bold and outgoing.

When we feel
Dull and ugly
You make us
Interesting and beautiful

When we feel
Ordinary and unsure
You make us
Extraordinary and confident

When we feel
Boring and trapped
You make us
Exciting and free!

Thank You
Jesus Christ
I Know
You are
My Lord
and Saviour.

©JEM 5am 21st June 2014

Matthew 28:18-20 (The Message)
18-20 Jesus, undeterred, went right ahead and gave his charge: "God authorized and commanded me to commission you: Go out and train everyone you meet, far and near, in this way of life, marking them by baptism in the threefold name: Father, Son, and Holy Spirit. Then instruct them in the practice of all I have commanded you. I'll be with you as you do this, day after day after day, right up to the end of the age."

Inspired from a conference encouraging us to invite those around us to join us following Our Lord Jesus Christ

Come Join With Me

Come
Join with me
Meet Jesus Christ
Love and give
Your life to Him.

Following Jesus
Is
the only way
You can be
truly happy
Each and every day.

He will lovingly
Guide you
Each and every
step of the way.

As you
follow Jesus
Doing work
for Him
Around
and within

You will
surely find
Fountains
of pure love
Torrents
of forgiveness
Waterfalls
of blessings

Following Jesus
Each step
of the way
Each and
every day

Is the
only way
To be forever
surrounded
By countless
blessings
each and every day.

© JEM 15th June 2014

<u>Matthew 4:19</u> NIVUK
   "Come, follow me," Jesus said, "and I will send you out to fish for people."

Inspired by a message that we all have a story to tell those who don't yet know about Our Lord Jesus Christ.

A Story to Tell

When Our Lord
Jesus Christ
Had a story to tell
He would sit down
with one or two
or even a crowd

He then would
Tell a story or two
So all there
That day
Would know
How His love
to others show.

He expects us
On others
His Love
to pour out

Telling our stories
Of how amazing
the love is that
He's given us

Leaving them
In no doubt
What He is all about.

They too will then
Catch hold of His love
and start following Him
Discovering how
His love really
fits life like a glove

Others then
will give friends
a shout telling them
what our Lord Jesus
is all about.

©JEM 6am 24th June 2014

Mathew 13:10-12 (The Message)

The disciples came up and asked, "Why do you tell stories?"He replied, "You've been given insight into God's kingdom. You know how it works. Not everybody has this gift, this insight; it hasn't been given to them. Whenever someone has a ready heart for this, the insights and understandings flow freely. But if there is no readiness, any trace of receptivity soon disappears. That's why I tell stories: to create readiness, to nudge the people toward receptive insight.

Inspired when I was reflecting on how many people have been blessed by my poetry once I gave in and joined social media. Posting the poems My Lord inspired me to write on facebook regularly.

Lord Sometimes We are so Slow

Lord sometimes
We are so slow
To embrace
what You
want us to know

Lord sometimes
We are so slow
To grab hold
Of the task
That we have
By You
been given

Lord sometimes
We are so slow
Your love to others
Down here below

Lord sometimes
You must despair

Why to others
we are so slow
To share your care
To those
about us everywhere.

Lord
Thank You
You are so patient
With us
Lord please help us
To quickly take up
The tasks You have
Already set us.

Lord help us
To straight away
Start looking for
The people
You want us to show
Your love and care to
Everyday.

©JEM 6am 25 June 2014

Matthew 9:37-38 (NIV)
Then he said to his disciples, "The harvest is plentiful but the workers are few.

Ask the Lord of the harvest, therefore, to send out workers into his harvest field."

This poem is a reflection of how God looked after me during the very tough years after my disabled son's birth.

Troubles

When life's troubles are
too massive a task,
He'll catch you!
Along the troubled pathway,
He'll carry you!

When it seems
too hard to keep going,
He'll cradle you!
When He calls
loved ones home,
He'll comfort you!

Jesus cares,
He's always here
Catching, carrying,
Cradling, and comforting
All those who ask Him.

Looking back,
glimpses He's given me of;
Where He's caught me,
When He's carried me,
Where He's cradled me,
When He's comforted me.

Where He's caught you,
When He's carried you,
Where He's cradled you,
When He's comforted you.
Will be plain to see,
When at last
life's work is done
And He's called you home
to sit on His knee.

Onward I go,
though trouble and woe
May visit me. I know,
He's always there, And one day,
I'll sit on His knee
My Jesus and me!

Hebrews 13:5 (The Message)
    Don't be obsessed with getting more material things. Be relaxed with what you have. Since God assured us, "I'll never let you down, never walk off and leave you," we can boldly quote, God is there, ready to help; I'm fearless no matter what. Who or what can get to me?

*Inspired by the different pathways and degrees of steepness &
speed of them God takes each of us on to continue His good work
right on time.*

The Staircase

Lord Jesus
A staircase you've set
for us to climb
No other is
the same as mine

Each staircase
You designed especially
To enable us
to climb it successfully

Each step requires
the best from us
Daily asking for
Your help a must!

Landings a plenty,
You put in place
So we can rest
then, renew the pace

When at last
we reach the top
Heaven's doors
will open pop.
And You will say
Welcome home
You're here to stay.

Psalm23 :1-3 (The Message)

God, my shepherd! I don't need a thing. You have bedded me down in lush meadows, You find me quiet pools to drink from. True to your word,

You let me catch my breath and send me in the right direction.

A reflection on some of the blessings we receive when we decide to ask Jesus Christ into our lives.

We are so Blessed

We are so blessed
Our Heavenly Father
Sent down His Son
So our freedom
Could be won.

We are so blessed
When day to day
life causes stress
Jesus replaces
That with rest

We are so blessed
When day to day
life gets us down
Jesus removes
our frown.

We are so blessed
When we ask
Jesus aboard
There is no test
We can't afford.

We are so blessed

Jesus removed
All our sins
When He died for us
Upon that tree
At Calvary

We are so blessed
To have Jesus
in our lives
they should display
Jesus every day

We are so blessed
We can others meet
To worship
Our Lord and
Our Saviour
At His Feet.

We are so blessed
We need to strive
To give Jesus
Our absolute best.

So I guess
you want so much
to join us
And be blessed

Give your life to
Jesus Christ
He will

Welcome, you in
so your life
blessed by Him
then can begin.

©JEM 4am 29th June 2014

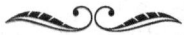

John 14:5-7 (The Message Bible)
5 Thomas said, "Master, we have no idea where you're going. How do you expect us to know the road?
"6-7 Jesus said, "I am the Road, also the Truth, also the Life. No one gets to the Father apart from me. If you really knew me, you would know my Father as well. From now on, you do know him. You've even seen him!"

Inspired, by a message on a Christian TV children's programme today.

You Ask Me Why

You ask me why
You should tell
Others about Jesus
Until His name
to them
rings like a bell

If Jesus hadn't come
No-one would love

If Jesus hadn't come
No-one would care

If Jesus hadn't come
No one would share

If Jesus hadn't come
No-one would give

If Jesus hadn't come
No-one would respect

If Jesus hadn't come
no-one would forgive

If Jesus hadn't come
No-one would be
Sin free.

If Jesus hadn't come
No-one could go to
Heaven.

So go tell everyone
Why Jesus did come.

©JEM 2pm 29th June 2014

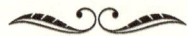

Psalm 138:8 GNT
You will do everything you have promised; Lord, your love is eternal.
Complete the work that you have begun.

A reflection back to His care for me when after the news at the antenatal appointment in What God Has Done For Me at the front of this book.

Lord Jesus You are My Everything

Lord Jesus,
You are
my everything
My Saviour,
my rescuer,
My carer,
my friend

The person in who
I can always trust
Telling others of this
is an absolute must!

MOST OF ALL
THAT NONE OF THIS
WILL EVER END!

Of You,
I will always;
others tell
Until, to them
Your name

rings like a bell
So they will
always know
THAT LIFE DOES NOT
NEED TO BE
A LIVING HELL.

You lifted me up
when I was down
Now, I never need
to wear a frown

I ONLY NEED
TO ASK
YOU FOR HELP

When into my life
Problems seem
to abound.
Lord Jesus
You show me
LOVE THAT HAS NO BOUNDS.

That day my life
was filled with fear
You Lord showed me
grace and care
To support me through
that day of fear

PEOPLE, JUST APPEARED,
FROM EVERYWHERE.

You, help me
So much
Throughout each day
You will, I know,
Keep others
from going astray

LORD SHOW ME
WHO YOU
NEED ME
TO HELP TODAY

Lord Jesus,
You are my king
Toyou,
I will always
praises sing;

THANK YOU LORD
FOR BEING MY EVERYTHING

©JEM 6 am, 6th August 2013

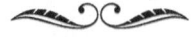

www.ingramcontent.com/pod-product-compliance
Lightning Source LLC
Chambersburg PA
CBHW030221140626
46545CB00011B/534